UNEXPECTED RESULTS

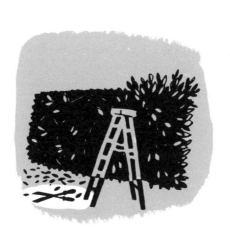

Unexpected Results

The Joy of Surgery

L. Newton Turk III, M.D.

FLATLINE PRESS

ATLANTA, GEORGIA

MMXIV

This book is printed on acid-free paper which conforms to the American National Standard z39.48.1984 Permanence of Paper for Printed Library Materials. Paper that conforms to this standard for pH, alkaline reserve, and freedom from groundwood is anticipated to last several hundred years without significant deterioration under normal library use and storage conditions.

Published by Flatline Press,
191 Peachtree Street, NE, Suite 4400, Atlanta, Georgia USA 30303.

First Edition
ISBN 978-0-615-92328-4
Printed in USA

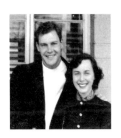

To Marcy

my wife and partner
in matters of the heart...
and to our children,
Susan, Julie, Bill, and Gregor.

Contents

Foreword

If there is one thing that equaled—or even exceeded—Newton Turk's passion for surgery, it was his passion for parenting. He loved playing as much as he loved working, and as father to his children, he knew well how to combine those two...how to find the balance between a demanding career and being present in the lives of four youngsters born in the span of six years' time.

We know that, of course, because we are those four children.

From our beginnings, we realized our dad was a surgeon. It was as much a part of him as his arms and legs. Even now, years after his retirement, we are approached by former patients, strangers to us who discover their surgeon is our dad. Some of those patients are so enthusiastic about the results of their experiences in the operating room with our dad at the helm that they grab our hand and place it over a scar or a slight rise of the skin on the chest under which rests the pacemaker our dad implanted there.

Most often these patients are convinced he saved their lives. We believe that, too. But when we tell our dad of those experiences, he recalls each case, remembers the patient's name, and says, "Oh, that was nothing...really."

Perhaps those cases were, in our dad's eyes, routine. But there were other cases that were not so routine, and whether he would admit to it or not, he did, indeed, save lives. This book highlights some of the cases Dad considered lifesavers.

We have heard bits and pieces of these cases from time to time, but here, these stories are fully told. And in their telling, we can see our dad at work in the O.R., we can hear his urgency in the situation, we can feel his adrenaline pumping, and most of all, we experience his joy.

"Oh that was nothing...really" was not false modesty. It was a heartfelt emotion expressed by a man who loved his job, who knew he could make a difference, who accepted the challenge, who delighted in unexpected results, and who bathed in the joy of it all.

That was the surgeon. And it is the dad, as well.

The two oldest of us remember living in New Haven, Connecticut, in an old duplex that backed up to the hospital parking lot. On any given morning, just as we were crawling out of bed, we would see our dad dashing across the parking lot from the hospital. He would be wearing white scrubs accented with red splashes of blood, a cotton surgical mask dangling from his pocket. He would come through the door, sit down at the table, eat a couple of fried eggs, kiss us goodbye and bound out the door, rushing back to the hospital as quickly as he had rushed in moments before.

By the time we moved to Kentucky, the scrubs had been replaced by a white coat with a stethoscope stuffed in the side pocket. Our house was scattered with piles of medical journals and surgical textbooks opened to various pages. Studying was his recreation.

On the occasions when Dad got home in time for dinner, he would usually plop down with the four of us—by then, our numbers had grown twofold—and in the middle of the living room floor, he would wrestle with us and toss us in the air. And then, almost in mid-toss, he would fall asleep. There he would stay, snoring soundly, until dinner was ready.

Dad stood six-feet, four-inches tall in his scrubs, but the size and gentleness of his larger-than-life hands is what we remember so well. At times the dining room table, draped in a solid cloth, would be covered in the brightly colored circuitry and wiring of a hi-fi system in mid-assemblage...a delicate operation of a different sort. We looked on in amazement at the complex, minute pieces Dad would surgically assemble to bring forth sound. Those same gifted hands built fine furniture over the years as well.

After we moved to Atlanta, Dad felt we were old enough to make rounds with him on the weekends. Trying to keep up with him in the hospital was a challenge. He rarely took the elevator, preferring to use the stairs as his mode of transportation. His long legs would climb them two or three at a time, and struggling behind him, we followed...our young legs working hard to catch up.

While he saw patients, we waited for him at the nurses' station, though on occasion we were allowed into rooms. Every now and then a patient would need a procedure, which meant we would be stuck at the hospital for hours. After enough of those experiences, we began to think long and hard before agreeing to go on rounds with him.

Here and there through our high school years, the only time we might see our dad during the week was when we heard his car in the driveway late at night after we had already gone to bed, and then again early in the morning when he left before dawn. We often pulled ourselves out of bed and watched from our windows just to get a glimpse of him.

It was also around this time that Dad invited us to watch operations. He would encourage us to include any of our friends who were interested in medicine. He was a stickler for proper operating room procedure, and we saw with our own eyes the surgeon, our dad, at his game...this man who made an undeniable contribution to the world of thoracic surgery as it took shape in Atlanta.

Obvious through it all was his passion for and his intensity in the intricacies of surgery. His whole demeanor as a surgeon was infectious. He absolutely loved what he did. It was clear to each of us that if we were ever patients requiring surgery, we would want those same qualities in our doctor.

Being there in the operating arena watching him work was an experience of a lifetime. All these years later, we still reflect on the indelible, treasured memory of our dad as he immersed himself in the joy of surgery, just as he immersed himself in the joy of being our dad.

Susan Turk Spratt
Julie Turk Martin
Bill Turk
Gregor Turk

2014

Preface

In February of the mid-seventies, a vascular surgeon friend of mine bought a new sailboat, a Morgan twenty-eight footer known as a Tiger Cub, to be precise. He invited me—along with three other physician friends—to crew the new boat in a two-day weekend race for the McNeil Cup on Lake Lanier in Georgia.

This was to be the captain's first race ever, as it was for each of the crew. We did not even know the names for the equipment on the boat or how to use any of it. With the exception of our captain, I may have been the only crew member who had ever sailed before...and that was on a sixteen-foot boat.

On the first race day, the competition rapidly narrowed to our boat and one other. That one was captained by Ted Turner who in 1977 won the America's Cup, you may recall. Anyway, our boat won the first day, and we were as surprised as the race watchers and our competition.

The second day was blustery and much colder. We got off to a good start only to find out quickly that we needed gloves to keep our hands anywhere near warm enough to be able to sail the ship. The only gloves we had were some thin rubber surgical gloves, which were worthless as hand warmers. Perhaps on this account, we were really in a hurry to finish the race and get warm again. Somehow we stayed out in front the whole way and thus won both halves of the event to take the McNeil Cup.

The sports headlines that followed in the local newspapers read something like this: "Green Physicians Win McNeil Cup."

Often we crew members have reminded each other about the sheer impossibility of having won. Occasionally, we have even had the opportunity to remind Ted as well.

Years have passed, and now we can barely remember the details of that day. What we do remember is the unmistakable feeling of having no chance to win, and therefore nothing to lose.

The lesson for three surgeons and one dermatologist, all with mighty cold hands, was something that would replay throughout our careers...the lesson of "unexpected results."

Introduction

I had always wanted to be a surgeon. I thought at first I wanted to practice general surgery, including chest, heart and vascular, and so I set out in that direction. But times were changing, and increasing specialization in narrowing areas was becoming the order of the day.

Nonetheless, my surgical training at Yale made me eligible to take both the general surgery and the thoracic surgery boards. The general surgery board was in two parts, written and oral. After that, one had to be certified by the general surgery board in order to be eligible to take the similar exams given by the Board of Thoracic Surgery. As soon as I was able to be scheduled for the examinations, I took them and passed them both. (For several years thereafter, I had occasional dreams in which I was taking some other board exam in a field for which I was not prepared and in which I was not trained, such as an internal medicine sub-specialty.)

During the years I spent in residency training and even afterwards, the nature of surgical practice changed drastically. By the early 1960s, general surgery and chest, heart and vascular surgeries were pretty much completely independent areas, and one did not have a chance to cross the boundaries anymore. In most metropolitan locations in the United States, the level of surgical specialization made it necessary to limit my field of endeavor and to become either a general surgeon, a thoracic surgeon, a heart surgeon, or a vascular surgeon. The general surgical training required a total of five years, and the thoracic training was one additional year. It has since increased to two years or more in some residency programs.

Counting four years in medical school, five years in general surgery training, and one to three years in thoracic and cardiovascular training, it now takes ten to thirteen years to become a fully trained thoracic surgeon.

I had been away from Atlanta where I was born and reared for about eleven years since graduating from undergraduate and medical school at Emory University in 1952. Most of those years away were spent learning general and thoracic surgery at Yale and Harvard in various capacities as an intern, resident, fellow and faculty member. Some of these positions were combined. For instance, at Harvard I was involved in a research fellowship and also held a humble faculty position. In all, I had sixty-six months of formal intern and resident training with a Yale faculty appointment during my eighteen months as chief resident there.

My wife, Marcy, worked hard at various hospital and medical school jobs while we were at Yale to supplement my internship pay, which amounted to a flat zero at that time. I can remember well how wonderful it was to rotate on the Veterans Administration Hospital surgical service where the residents got a small, but meaningful paycheck every two weeks.

I also spent a couple of years at Walker Air Force Base in New Mexico on active duty serving as a flight surgeon in the U.S. Air Force Reserve. I topped out as a major in 1956. The Air Force assignment was a golden opportunity at that stage in my preparation to be a surgeon. I had ready access to a well-qualified community of surgeons in various specialties to aid and comfort me, making it possible for me to safely grow my surgical skills.

I then became a practitioner of general and thoracic surgery and a part-time clinical faculty member at the newly opened University of Kentucky School of Medicine in Lexington.

The Lexington experience was interesting. There was a complete and distinguished surgical faculty, including Drs. Frank Spencer and Ben Eiseman, two of my favorite academic surgeons. But because the school was so new, there were no third- or fourth-year medical students, surgical interns or residents to be taught, and it was hard to know how best to expose first- and second-year students to surgery in a meaningful way. Surgery was usually a subject for the final two years of medical school when students had developed patient-care skills in other areas. We provided opportunities to do some animal operations, mainly because the surgical faculty just could not wait to teach somebody about operative surgery.

There were three residency programs in surgery in Lexington in 1960, and the three young surgeons who were there—of which I was one—provided most of the resident supervision and teaching for the three programs. From this experience, I learned that I liked being a private practitioner and a clinical teacher of surgical residents rather than being an academic surgeon.

Up to that time, general surgery had been truly general, and it included chest and cardiovascular. I remember fondly in Lexington when my first case of the day was a heart valve replacement in one patient followed by an operation for an ingrown toenail in another.

In big cities, though, times were changing. Surgeons were already moving into separate surgical specialty areas, and I would have to do the same.

When—after a little over two years in Lexington—an opportunity to join a chest and cardiovascular surgical practice in Atlanta turned up and seemed to provide just the situation I wanted, I took it.

Unlike most new doctors nowadays, I had borrowed only a small amount of money during my training years. With the help of my Air Force salary, a full dose of financial support from the G.I. Bill, and a couple of research fellowships that paid well, my school debts were few. By the time we moved to

Atlanta, I had already paid back my modest and only education debt, which was to my father-in-law.

Getting a practice off the ground was fortunately not a big problem. My family provided plenty of motivation. My dad was a physician in Atlanta for many years and had a number of physician friends who were willing to give me a chance to see what I could do. And what I could do was to be available and eager to go to any of the ten or so various hospital emergency rooms about town when called upon to see patients who were sick or injured and might need chest surgery.

Atlanta was becoming a major metropolis and growing rapidly when my family and I moved back in 1963. We had always wanted to be in Atlanta, and by this time, my hometown had shown it was serious about successfully integrating its public schools and proving it really was "a city too busy to hate." In fact, Atlanta's schools and public facilities were integrated without any big problems about eight months ahead of the National Civil Rights Act of 1964.

And so, reassured by the ease with which the Atlanta public schools had been integrated, especially compared to those in some other locations, we migrated there in the spring of '63. I was the sixth thoracic surgeon to come to Atlanta.

Buoyed by good schools, peaceful integration, an airport on its way to becoming internationally known, and local political leadership that was both strong and wise, Atlanta began a journey of weed-like growth. It would be a good place to practice medicine and rear our children.

We bought a new house in the northeastern part of town near Buckhead where there was a particularly strong public grammar school for the older two children. Together with some friends and neighbors, we helped start a Montessori school which our two pre-school children enjoyed. The school also provided the supporting parents with opportunities to maintain our painting and fix-up skills because we needed to have functional classroom space, which we borrowed at several different locations in church basements. We even borrowed some still-standing, World War II-era veterans' hospital buildings, meant only to be temporary when they were originally constructed. Basically, our custodial activities served as rent for the space we needed.

The school has been quite successful over the past thirty-five years or so, though it is now housed in a somewhat grander style on its own campus. Two of our children and three grandchildren have attended—and benefited—from the school. We firmly believe our painting and carpentry work have been richly rewarded. Over the years, we founding fathers and mothers of the First Montessori School of Atlanta (now Springmont) have been honored locally at various public celebrations as pioneer educators. Apparently, we have successfully managed to keep it a secret that we were essentially just a bunch of fix-up and clean-up volunteers.

As it has worked out, I have practiced chest surgery and have been involved with resident training in surgery for about forty-seven years in Atlanta. All those years ago, I arrived on the scene completely outfitted with a marvelous wife and four small children. I have since decided it was really near the height of hopeful self-confidence that would put together a family of six without visible means of support except for me—the new doctor in town.

UNEXPECTED RESULTS

CHAPTER ONE

Where have all the surgeons gone?

Increasingly, concern is being raised about a shortage of surgeons in the United States, which may turn out to be difficult or impossible to avoid and/or correct. The shortage is said to already be apparent in some of the more rural and thinly populated areas of the country such as Alaska. The problem seems to be related both to fewer medical graduates choosing to be surgeons and to mature surgeons who are deciding to limit their working time or to quit practicing surgery altogether. Other multiple factors also play a role in this problem, which include poorly informed Congressional and bureaucratic regulatory activity, the long period of preparation and training to be a surgeon, excessive and changing government regulations, insufficient and slow payment for services, a large and perhaps inconvenient burden of trauma, long duty hours, debt residuals from training and medical school, and out-of-control litigation.

Interestingly enough, until quite recently government planners were concerned that too many physicians were being trained, especially in the subspecialties of medicine as well as in most of the surgical arenas. Consequently, these planners advised changing the amounts of money contributed by government for resident training support mainly through the Medicare program. This, they thought, would prevent what they saw as an oversupply of surgeons. More general family medicine providers were thought to be the answer, and the output and training of these physicians was encouraged and increased. Some policymakers seem to be of the opinion that there are now more family doctors than are needed and maybe not enough surgical specialists. It seems we have yet to strike the right balance.

Several new medical schools began operation in the 1960s and '70s just as some of the established schools of medicine were beginning to increase the number of their students, all in an effort to provide an adequate total number of physicians. The health planners were left to predict what the right number of doctors would be for the different medical and surgical specialties.

The bureaucrats, using assumptions since proved to be well off the mark, also fixed caps on the numbers of residents for whom teaching hospitals would be able to collect training fees. This limited the number of residents who could be trained as surgeons and the various types of surgical specialists, leading in part to the passage of the Balanced Budget Act of 1997[1]. It was a poorly informed United States Congress which placed further restrictions on the number of surgeons who could be trained.

In 1994, indicators for general surgery showed that 1,874 trainees attempted to match in the National Resident Matching Plan (NRMP) for the 1,133 general surgical categorical Postgraduate Year One training positions available. In 2007, only 1,057 categorical surgical training positions were available and 1,043 graduating medical students seeking to match for training. In the latest NRMP for cardiothoracic surgery, there were ninety-four applicants for the 118 available positions.

It is clear that fewer medical students want to be surgeons now, a path that takes five to seven years beyond medical school. And even though there are more and more women becoming physicians, not as many of them want to go into surgery as have men up to now.

Recertification in the various specialties is another fairly recent change in the requirements of practicing physicians that is principally protective of patients. It seems to be a potential deterrent for some career pathways, but it is doubtful any significant change in this area is likely other than further refinements in the evaluation process for certification renewals.

In addition, surveys of presently practicing surgeons recently show that many have a desire to retire from the profession when they feel able to do so, if present conditions prevail. The current practitioners of surgery in the United States include an increasing number who are fifty-five years of age or older. They may soon be in a position to seriously consider retirement or perhaps no longer practice surgery at all. They might opt for some modification of their work activities that allows them to cut back on their surgical workload. This could include downgrading to a less demanding work schedule or a different type of activity such as no longer taking trauma calls or performing other tasks that are personally unacceptable at that stage in their careers. The lifestyle of the general surgeon and many of the surgical sub-specialists is for the most part more demanding than that of many other specialties, and the monetary rewards at present are not always commensurate with the efforts required.

Medicare has effectively fixed prices for many of the surgeon's activities, and there is much concern about threatened reductions in the reimbursement levels for some procedures, especially those performed by general surgeons. The level of uncertainty created by Medicare policy and payment changes is also a potential major deterrent for those considering a career as a general surgeon. Remunerations by Medicare and/or other insurance providers to hospitals and surgeons who are on emergency room call and who must be in the hospital overnight is also presently facing considerable opposition.

So who wants to become a general surgeon now? Obviously, not as many as have wanted to in the past.

The American College of Surgeons, the dominant professional association for various kinds of surgeons, is encouraging its members and leadership to consider changes in the training process now being followed. This might head off a surgical shortage and provide adequate numbers of surgeons to handle our growing elderly population.

The essence of surgical training is found in the one year (or more) of chief resident responsibilities that are strictly required for Board eligibility. In my case, there were eighteen months at this level, and at that time there was no limit on the number of hours per week the chief or any other resident could put in. Since 2003, the Accreditation Council for Graduate Medical Education (ACGME) has put a limit of eighty hours per week on resident work and duty hours.

Having been in the accreditation business as the eighty-hour-per-week duty limitation was imposed, I believe it is a good thing and probably should have been in place long before it was actually implemented. Even with mixed reviews from some surgical educators and program directors, this does seem to be a step in the right direction, though it is doubtful it will be enough by itself to solve the problem. There are those who believe the educational process suffers when confined to eighty hours per week, yet there are others who are discussing the practicality of a sixty-hour maximum for resident hours per week.

The other main step in making surgeons a happier lot is the emergence of surgical "hospitalists" who take responsibility for in-patient treatment for limited, scheduled periods of time. They also perform emergency surgery and take care of much of the surgical workload, especially during after-hours. It is undecided how this will affect the popularity of becoming either a surgical hospitalist/traumatologist with regular hours and regular time off or of being a busy surgeon who does almost exclusively elective cases without dealing much with emergencies and trauma. One way to put these together is to be the hospitalist on certain days and the elective surgeon at other times, effectively forming a group practice of sorts with other like-minded individuals.

Surgical techniques and technology are changing at an increasingly rapid rate. The paperwork aspect of medicine is now computerized. This should affect the surgeon directly and improve productivity across the board.

The pay during residency training has improved significantly throughout the years. In my own case, it went from zero as an intern to the princely sum of about three hundred dollars per month as chief resident. Since my training days, pay has now come close to a living wage, though not to a level that usually allows much of a chance at debt reduction. Still, the rewards of surgery are great in ways that have nothing to do with payment for services.

Around the time my surgical career began, I looked on the prospects of becoming a surgeon the way I imagine astronaut candidates look on their hopes of being selected for the job. I thought surgery, particularly in those days when there were such rapid advances in cardiac surgery, was an astronaut-like opportunity and that nothing else compared to it except perhaps being the king of a small to medium–sized country. I am greatly concerned that this kind of feeling for a career in surgery has somehow lost its popularity and appeal among the young people who are making a career choices today. Perhaps something I could point out about surgery within these pages might cast things in a different light. That is my hope.

CHAPTER TWO

The Joy of Surgery

When viewed over the course of a career, there may be—and often are—clearly enjoyable experiences interspersed with the hard work, late hours and diminished family interaction that typify the usual medical practice, especially the practice of surgery. The source of much of the enjoyment is tied to patient interactions and the achievement of personal and professional satisfaction during the surgical care process. This feeling is multiplied when the course of events during recovery indicates the results may be turning out far better than anyone had a right to expect.

The stories included in this book are of a handful of patients and situations over my thirty-plus years of practice as a thoracic surgeon. They serve to express the idea that there can be unexpected results, which bring great joy from the practice of surgery.

The joy of surgery has nothing to do with any kind of reimbursement, but everything to do with an immense sense of accomplishment that comes with surgical success. The cases included in this book were of great difficulty when rapid decision-making was necessary and success was unpredictable and often doubtful.

I have selected a small group of eight seriously challenged patients with a variety of traumatic and other near-fatal conditions who had the good grace to respond favorably to my management of their problems. All required major chest surgery, and all were fortunate enough to get well when it appeared certain the chances were against them.

As you might imagine, when other ex-patients discover they are not among the select eight, they often want to know why they did not make the cut. Some of them have assumed, sometimes correctly, that they also have been saved by thoracic surgery. I tell them they were too well behaved and did not challenge my skill level to the maximum.

The ones who were selected are in no way your average run-of-the-mill cases. These patients were chosen for inclusion here because of their unexpected results, and consequently, they are known to me familiarly as "specials." Their stories are all true, but the names and a few identifying factors have been changed to protect the privacy of these good folks. All of them experienced conditions and circumstances which made survival unlikely, and all had to overcome unfavorable-to-overwhelming odds in order to survive.

Furthermore, to qualify as specials, these patients had to get well when the chances for recovery were poor to abysmal, and a successful outcome in each case was beyond rational expectations. Even Joe, Brian and Fred, the three specials diagnosed with cancer, got well and have remained well for over two decades.

I do not plan to go into a lot of detail about technical matters and medical mumbo-jumbo, at least nothing I can't give the sense of with a well-placed parenthetical aside. I do not plan to dwell on the disease processes of these patients overmuch, but rather on the patients themselves as much as possible. I have tried to select a sort of cross-section of some of the most serious dilemmas a thoracic surgeon faces, but the unvarying characteristic throughout all eight stories is that of a happy ending.

This is a feel-good kind of presentation, and there is no apology coming for that. There is grief and trouble aplenty in the thoracic surgery business, and that part of it will be left for others to tell. This will deal only with excellent and positive outcomes.

The stories are not primarily about a doctor, or about a few specific serious disease processes, or even about chest surgery in general, but about a small group of people who happened to have had serious challenges to their survival during certain illnesses or after certain accidents. Each patient's problem turned out to be amenable to surgery. All decisions as to treatment and procedure were mine, and I performed all of the surgeries during a period from 1958 to 1988.

My estimate for the odds of a favorable outcome for these patients was from about twenty-five percent in the most favorable cases to less than five percent for others. Current literature puts the chance of survival from a spontaneously ruptured esophagus, for example, at less than ten percent and from a traumatic rupture of the thoracic aorta at about twenty percent or less. Most of these result in immediate death.

I am not claiming any special skill or knowledge beyond that of any well-trained and experienced chest surgeon. I state only that I did my best for each patient with the available knowledge and tools to overcome the problems presented.

Since the practice of a chest surgeon in the last forty years has been so largely involved with lung cancer, questions might arise among readers about the lack of any patients with that particular problem in this group. I can only say that lung cancer in my practice just did not provide any patients with the immediate life or death potentials of the likes of bloody arterial injuries, a smelly torn esophagus, or a hedge-clipped heart.

These specials are truly survivors and have all provided this surgeon with powerful feelings of accomplishment and thankfulness to have participated in the management of their problems.

I take great pleasure in friendly association, from time to time, with my former patients including the specials, all of whom are long-term survivors of conditions they were not expected to overcome. Each of them had unexpected results. To me, it is a small indication of the personal satisfaction that comes from the opportunities provided in what I consider "The Joy of Surgery."

CHAPTER THREE

The Specials

ROSA DOESN'T DRINK COFFEE ANYMORE

REVEREND CHARLES

GEORGE, WHO FELL ON HIS SWORD

A SURPRISE GOING-AWAY PRESENT FROM DELORES

SAM AND THE LONG, LONG, LONG TUNNEL

JOE PREPARES FOR A RACE WITH CANCER

BRIAN AND FRED—HOW DID THAT HAPPEN?

All of the specials had similar kinds of adventures in "chest surgery land" under my care. Their problems were responsive to the surgical procedures and surgical care I was able to carry out. They all got well from their various complex problems and all had happy endings, though the happy endings may have been unanticipated and were certainly not guaranteed. In the situations in which they were involved, the odds for success ranged from not good to terrible.

Having current access to some of the folks in this small but unusual group of former patients led me to try to determine what, if any, effect their surgical experiences may have had on their subsequent lives and whether having such experiences changed their outlook, beliefs or chosen activities. Each of the specials has had ample opportunity to examine the implications or purpose of his or her survivorship.

While each has come to understand well that he or she is indeed in a special situation, so far no demands have been placed on them to do anything recognizable as any sort of a mission. For the most part, the specials I have talked with have had little impression that they were saved for some specific purpose or that they will be called upon to do something or other as payment for their survival.

By fortunate accident, it has worked out that I have maintained at least some social contact with many of these folks after my retirement from active practice. The place where my wife and I live is on one of the barrier islands on the coast of Georgia. Here, twenty-five to perhaps thirty other former patients or their families also live. Among them are several of the specials with whom my wife and I have had social contact on an ongoing basis. I can certainly attest to the fact that it does not hurt to have folks like these as fervent supporters in the community and on my side no matter what.

As I have worked on this book, I have gotten some updated information about others of the specials from various sources, but even Google does not know where some of them are hanging out now. The good thing is that several of them have been located, and I have followed up in an informational fashion. Others have not been in contact for twenty years or more.

Much of the attention these days about unexpected human survival relates to the near-death kinds of incidents such as cardiac arrest. This kind of event usually includes a partial or complete loss of consciousness due to a temporary lack of adequate oxygenation or flow of blood. This may leave the patient with some memory loss or altered perceptions of events which have gone on during the period of oxygen deprivation.

The specials generally were not subjected to that kind of insult, but rather had a more or less planned surgical operation under anesthesia in a hospital environment. They did not, for the most part, have a lack of oxygen as the main cause of their problems, though there undoubtedly was some oxygenation difficulty intermittently in Sam's case. Subsequent events did not suggest any identifiable residual deficits that might be attributed to a lack of oxygenation. Even the patient whose major arterial sources of oxygenated blood to the head and brain had to be ligated in order to control the bleeding did not suffer from a lack of oxygenation.

The patients described in this account—including Sam—did not report any of the kinds of near-death experiences that would be ascribed to a critical lack of oxygen. Their problems were generally of a different order of magnitude.

A good part of the reason I am describing this material through my writing, aside from reminding myself of pleasant times, is to attract young people to consider a surgical career. Although there are some problems and difficulties in any

medical or surgical career these days, these true stories—
subject always to the imperfections in the memories of those
involved—are aimed to show the shiny side of surgery from a
chest surgeon's point of view. I look upon these stories as what
surgeons would like to have happen every time they pick up a
knife to work on a patient.

My first special is Rosa, from my residency days in 1958. The
others are, in essence, the rest of my "Rosas," collected over a
career in chest surgery. Each special challenged my skills as a
surgeon and produced a feel-good reaction for me.

In Rosa's story, there is also the opportunity to see an
example of a major change in procedural technique, moving
from open-chest massage to the far better technique of closed-
chest cardiac massage. This was done with ample scientific
investigation, proving that the change was justified and
advantageous. A standard protocol is being provided today for
anybody who is interested in gaining the ability to do cardiac
resuscitation even single-handedly.

Generally, surgery is a science that is always in a state of
change as better and more effective ways of doing things are
developed. Surgical residents no longer carry a sterile scalpel,
and patients no longer have to fear waking up with somebody's
hand in their chest, squeezing their heart.

Robotic surgery is another area of great change, especially
with a refinement of laparoscopic procedures (minimally
invasive surgery) that have been developing over the past

several years. The full influence of this type of innovation on the practice of surgery is yet to be determined, along with its effect on the supply of surgeons, but it is expected to decrease the time required to perform various operative procedures, especially those in the chest and abdomen.

While surgical techniques continue to change and improve, the human rewards remain as is. That I was able to return Rosa to her children was particularly important to me. It continues to be something I treasure. It has made all the hard work and long hours demonstrably worthwhile.

Rosa Doesn't Drink Coffee Anymore

The voice was clearly agitated as it came over the public address system. The year was 1958, and the place was Grace-New Haven Community Hospital, later renamed the Yale-New Haven Hospital, in New Haven, Connecticut. It is the principal teaching hospital for the Yale School of Medicine.

The one being paged by name was me. The codes told me the problem and the place: cardiac arrest; emergency room.

I had just assumed the position of chief cardiovascular surgery resident at Yale and was the physician who was designated to respond and be the team leader during such an event. I rushed to the emergency clinic area, taking the four flights of stairs downward two or three steps at a time. I then reminded myself that if I fell down the stairs and became injured in the fall, I would hardly be helpful to either the patient or myself. It is funny how useless information like that gets remembered sometimes, even when there is a high level of current excitement, as in this instance. Anyway, I still recall that trip down the stairs and my sudden fractional increase in caution and use of the handrails.

I whizzed into the emergency room and found a young woman unconscious on a stretcher. She was being given oxygen through a face mask, and her lungs were being inflated regularly. She was wired for electrocardiogram monitoring, but it showed only a straight line with no heartbeats. I gave a quick listen with a stethoscope and a swift feel for a pulse in her neck without finding any signs of life. I followed what protocol there was at the time, which was to give a whack with the hand over the heart. Nothing happened. Then I pulled out the ever-present sterile scalpel that I and many other surgery residents carried in a glass vial in our pockets for just such an occasion.

This was my first opportunity to have the experience and responsibility as team leader for a cardiac resuscitation. In those days, it was always performed by opening the patient's left chest and doing manual cardiac massage "open technique" by squeezing the patient's heart gently but firmly about once per second. I understandably wanted the outcome to be successful for my first exposure in the decision maker's role.

With the diagnosis satisfactorily confirmed, we turned the patient partially on her right side, and I made a rapid incision in the left chest underneath the breast. The heart was completely still as it came into view, and holding the ribs apart with one hand, I began to carry out cardiac massage, rhythmically squeezing and relaxing. When I could manage to see the heart in all this process, it was still clearly not beating. Meanwhile, others saw to the inflation and deflation of her lungs using a face mask, a rubber bag, and a flow of oxygen.

After about ten or fifteen minutes of massage and oxygenation, her heart started beating again. She became fully awake and was obviously in a lot of pain. This was taken as a positive development and reason to be encouraged about success. Assuming the operating room I had requested was ready, we took our patient there, and an anesthesiologist gave her some anesthetic for pain relief. After a period of further observation during which her heart continued beating regularly, her blood pressure returned to normal. I then set about to close the incision. Her heart continued to beat in regular fashion, and she began to awaken from the anesthetic as we moved her to the recovery room for close observation.

During the ensuing days following surgery, it became apparent Rosa had not suffered any brain damage or any other significant sequelae from her arrest. Over the course of the next week or so, Rosa made a progressive and quite satisfactory recovery.

It turned out she was extremely sensitive to caffeine, and on that fateful morning with her friends, Rosa had enjoyed several cups of coffee, which was not her usual habit. After drinking the coffee, she had collapsed and passed out several times at home and again in the emergency room, but on that last occasion, her heart did not start beating again. Her problem was rapidly diagnosed and remedied in the emergency room, thanks to the alertness of the hospital staff.

Rosa had been in good health and was the mother of two small, precious children. She left the hospital in good shape, and as far as I know, never drank any more coffee.

I had a powerful feeling of gratitude because I had been able to handle the situation well, the resuscitation had been successful, and I had been able to save Rosa's young children from a life without their mother. Rosa was, after all, the first opportunity I had been offered to save a life and accomplish the kind of thing I had been working hard and long to do as a surgeon. I also had a feeling of pride and accomplishment that I found pleasant, and I hoped I would be able to have it again in future successful surgical adventures.

Rosa seemed to be fully restored to her pre-arrest condition and had no significant problems or residuals during the eighteen months I remained in contact with her before I left New Haven.

I had completed a study during an earlier part of my training regarding Yale's experience with cardiac arrest. I published an account in the November 1954 issue of the *New England Journal of Medicine*[2] about seven successful resuscitations in forty-five cases of cardiac arrest over a five-year period ending in 1954. That report and study, combined with the success of

Rosa's case pretty much made me the local expert in cardiac arrest, which did not hurt in the highly competitive world of surgery.

The technique I used to resuscitate Rosa, open-chest cardiac massage, was supplanted within a few short years by the discovery that closed-chest massage was just about equally effective. As I have mentioned, it is now the technique of choice by far because it does not require any incision, can be done by anybody who learns it, and does not need any special equipment.

Rosa was the first patient I had who was clearly a "saved life" due to my efforts and the efforts of others as well. I realized there were any number of ways it could have turned out differently—like if I had fallen down the stairs or had not been sure there was no heartbeat. Anyhow, Rosa's two kids got to keep their mom, and I learned some useful things that better prepared me to face other similar circumstances.

Reverend Charles

Some summers, I would have a sophomore or junior medical student spend time with me in order to see what a surgical practice is like. I paid a token small salary and enjoyed having an avid learner with me at the office, in the hospital, and in the operating room.

This particular summer, a student named Paul was with me. A keen observer, Paul would go on to become a surgical subspecialist with a highly successful career as a urologist. Before our summer together was over, Paul commissioned an artist friend to paint an operating room scene as a gift to me. I hung it proudly in my office and even made a logo version of it to use in my slide presentations.

The evening I first met the man we will refer to as Reverend Charles, Paul was having dinner at my house. We were just finishing dessert when there was an urgent call from one of the university hospitals. A patient was in the emergency room having really severe, apparently non-cardiac, chest pain. This patient's family doctor was with him.

Even though he was not on duty after suppertime, Paul wanted to be involved to see what this pain was all about.

I told him my over-the-phone diagnosis was Boerhaave Syndrome, a spontaneous rupture of the esophagus first described in 1724 by a famous Dutch physician, Dr. Herman Boerhaave (1668-1738).

Watch out. A little medical history is coming at you.

Boerhaave Syndrome usually follows a heavy meal and some vomiting, but occasionally may be associated with a head injury followed by nausea and vomiting and having nothing to do with a meal or anything eaten.

Dr. Boerhaave attended the Dutch Grand Admiral, Baron Jan Gerrit van Wassenaer, a well-known trencherman who experienced sudden, severe chest pains and began vomiting after a wonderfully large meal that included roast duck. The grand admiral died within hours, and Dr. Boerhaave then carried out an autopsy. He was immediately aware of a strong odor of roast duck when he opened the admiral's chest, indicating there was some kind of a tear between the esophagus and the chest cavity. The odor immediately suggested to Dr. Boerhaave that there was an esophageal rupture, and that is, of course, exactly what was found. Dr. Boerhaave's detailed and classic description of the cogent findings, written in Latin, filled over seventy pages and resulted in spontaneous esophageal rupture being called the Boerhaave Syndrome from that time forward.

Other observations in more recent times have shown that the mortality rate of the condition relates strongly to the time between the rupture and diagnosis. About twenty-five percent of patients die during the passage of the first twelve hours; sixty-five percent during the first twenty-four hours; eighty-nine percent by forty-eight hours; and a hundred percent by the end of one week according to a report about this syndrome.

Obviously the problem needs to be quickly diagnosed and the esophagus repaired as soon as possible. The first written report of a successful surgical repair of a spontaneous esophageal rupture did not appear in the surgical literature until 1946. Fortunately, it is a rare occurrence and one that is relatively easy to diagnose accurately.

During the dessert-time call from the hospital, I asked for a limited esophagram to be performed while Paul and I drove to the hospital. A limited esophagram is an X-ray of the esophagus after the patient swallows a small amount of a contrast substance. If there is a rupture of the esophagus, it is readily apparent on the X-ray when the contrast material collects in the chest cavity due to the esophageal tear. I suspected this would be the finding. I told Paul this problem was a serious one and that it demanded surgical repair of the esophagus as quickly as possible.

In our situation, about 275 years after Dr. Boerhaave's experience with the grand admiral, Reverend Charles' esophagram confirmed the diagnosis and showed a lower esophageal tear with spillage of the contrast material into the chest cavity. This was now a confirmed textbook case with all the usual Boerhaave characteristics, except for the roast duck aroma. All we had to do was fix the leakage of eaten material into the chest, get the esophagus to heal, and control and abate the infection in the chest due to the leaked stomach and esophageal contents there.

Charles was a man of about fifty who had enjoyed generally good health and was the senior minister in one of the large suburban Atlanta churches. Because of his severe chest pain, Charles and his family, along with his personal doctor, were all in favor of my immediate recommendation to take prompt action to repair the damaged esophagus. Without question, this would provide him with the best and really only chance for survival and recovery.

Paul was delighted to be part of the team and to see how the patient, the family, and the referring physician were all involved in the decisions which were made in this most urgent and serious situation. This kind of exposure and on-scene involvement for a medical student, especially one contemplating a surgical career, provides some of the best teaching and learning opportunities, though for some reason, these opportunities seem to be most prevalent after dark and on weekends.

We went straight to the operating room, and with Charles under general anesthesia, we opened the left chest and found the expected tear of the lower esophagus. A careful repair of the esophagus was followed by placing sutures in the esophagus to seal the torn area. The chest cavity was irrigated—washed out—thoroughly with saline solution to remove as much of the swallowed material as possible. The patient remained stable through the procedure and tolerated it well. I estimated we had a good chance for recovery since we were still within the first four hours of the onset of the rupture.

Reverend Charles had a somewhat rocky recovery and spent several days in the intensive care unit. He was being given some heavy-duty pain medications and generous doses of intravenous antibiotics to overcome the infection in the chest cavity. Charles had some periods of mental confusion during his stay in the intensive care unit, but it quickly became clear that his esophagus was in healing mode. He was eventually moved from intensive care to a regular hospital room, and the confusion disappeared as he came off the heavy pain-relief medications. At the end of about two weeks, Charles was without any fever, swallowing well, and was getting up and about with more and more ease. He was indeed ready to go home for further convalescence.

Charles continued to improve, regain his strength, and increase his activity level toward its normal range at home. Paul and I followed him in the office on several visits, and his recovery continued in uneventful fashion.

I felt that Charles' own family doctor had contributed
materially to our success since he had realized the seriousness
of Charles' situation right away. He also aided in moving Paul
and me forward to proceed quickly with confirmation of the
diagnosis and to get the surgery underway as rapidly as possible.
The hospital staff had also risen to the occasion in wonderful
style and provided all the support we required.

Paul was glad to have been in on the whole process from
start to finish and to see how emergency surgery can be
exciting sometimes, especially when all goes well.

One day several months later, long after Paul was back in
medical school and unavailable to me, I got an invitation from
a physician friend to attend services at Reverend Charles'
church. I was sorry Paul was not able to be there because he
had taken a real interest in Charles' recovery, but my wife and
I felt we should attend the service. I soon realized it would
have been far better had I been able to get Paul there instead of
being there myself.

I was totally unprepared for the morning's events as
Reverend Charles started what I assumed would be his sermon.
He asked me to stand up, and instead of a usual sermon for
his parishioners, he went through a glowing description of his
recent hospital experiences and how he owed his life to me
and to Paul. Some of the things he described as having gone

on in the early days of his hospitalization were, in part at least, contributed to by some of the medications he was receiving at that time. He may have been telling some of his narcotic-influenced dreams. In any event, I was thoroughly embarrassed, and after the sermon, I got to spend a half hour meeting and shaking hands with Charles' grateful congregation.

I felt like telling the congregation that most of what Charles had said was the narcotics talking and that I was not really half as wonderful as he had claimed. Upon reflection, though, I did not think I should tell the good folks that a lot of what Charles had said was probably just some narco-speak from those first few days after the operation.

I told Paul later what had happened and that if he were ever in the same position, my advice was not to accept any invitations to go to churches where he had treated the preacher successfully unless he was prepared to be seriously embarrassed. Of course, Charles did not mean to embarrass me. He was just a grateful patient who felt he should be thankful in public as well as in private.

Charles was one of three Boerhaave Syndrome cases that were referred to me for surgery in a short space of time fairly soon after I began practice in Atlanta. Fortunately, all three got well, and I had something to use as lecture material that was unusual, interesting, local and successful. I seemed to have become the esophagus guy in town for a while.

Charles resumed his duties as a pastor for his flock for several years. He then had other assignments until his death in the mid '90's from an unknown cause, apparently unrelated to his esophagus.

Needless to say, I thought of Reverend Charles every time I drove by his church, even long after he was no longer the pastor there.

George, Who Fell on his Sword

We rarely get the chance to treat people who fall on their own swords as the ancient Romans and others did when they became irremediable losers in battle or total failures at something important in life. This story is about an accidental, rather than a purposeful, sword-falling episode which did not involve a sword at all but a sword-like, common, hand-powered hedge clipper.

It happened to a young man who was certainly no failure. We will call him George. His wife, who is prominent in the story, will be Mary.

George was a healthy young executive who was about six-feet tall and a former B-26 pilot. He and Mary were newly arrived in Atlanta after a job promotion and an increase in his responsibilities. He was achieving district manager status in a large manufacturing corporation and had moved into a new house in a nice part of Atlanta just a few weeks earlier.

On that pleasant early spring Saturday afternoon, George was trying to be helpful around the couple's new house and volunteered to trim a tall hedge that Mary could not quite reach. He was using a pair of big, old, hand-operated hedge shears because neither he nor Mary could find their brand-new, electric-powered hedge trimmer which had gotten lost in the shuffle of the move.

George was in the process of trimming the high part of the hedge and was changing his location, carrying the ladder and clippers. Suddenly and unexpectedly, as he was about to climb the ladder, one of his feet became tangled in a small wire fence hidden in the shrubbery and grass. George lost his balance, falling forward heavily. As he was falling, he dropped the tools he was carrying, but he was unable to keep himself from falling. The handles of the clippers hit the ground first and stuck in the debris there so that the clipper blade pointed skyward. George fell chest-first right onto the business end of one of the clipper blades. The long, sharply pointed blade impaled itself straight into the middle of his lower chest, right about where the mammalian heart resides.

George experienced a lot of pain and a lot of bleeding. Mary immediately recognized she had a difficult problem and a serious situation.

Fortunately for George, Mary was a wife whose most important attribute at that moment was a cool head. She possessed the ability to adapt to a serious situation and to function impressively without becoming flustered or upset.

Mary asked a neighbor to contact the closest hospital to prepare them for George's arrival which was expected to be no more than twenty minutes. She must get George to the hospital, and she would do it by car.

But George was not able to fit in the car doorway due to the protruding clipper blade. He took care of this problem by grabbing the offending clipper handle and pulling what he later estimated was about six inches of clipper blade out of his chest. He was then able to get into the car. He positioned himself inside the car, and quickly discovered that without the blade in his chest, he could diminish the bleeding by compressing the wounded area with his hands and pulling his legs firmly against his chest.

My home was only about ten to fifteen minutes from Piedmont Hospital, and especially in my early years of practice, I was eager to have a chance to see emergencies and all sorts of chest injuries. I would be called sometimes, like in this instance, because the emergency room nurses knew I lived close by, and I would come try to take care of a problem even when I was not assigned to be on call to the hospital's emergency room.

And so, the hospital emergency room nurse telephoned me and explained George's situation. I asked them to get the operating room and anesthesia crews ready for surgery as quickly as they could. She rounded up a surgical team of nurses and an emergency room intern, got the anesthesiologist and the anesthetic equipment together, and prepared the surgical tools we would need.

Mary and George were already on their way to the hospital, but their trip was a nightmare and took close to fifty minutes because of the unusually heavy traffic. Their progress was slowed by cars going in and out of a huge shopping center. Mary kept blowing the car horn, but people showed little interest in pulling over and letting her go by. Atlanta traffic still seems to contain a lot of those same drivers.

George was now looking pretty weak and pale, and he was having a hard time maintaining the pressure to slow the bleeding. He also began to feel his extremities growing cold. Mary said later that although George was the color of putty, he never lost consciousness and remained able to staunch the bleeding from his chest wound as much as possible on the long trip to the hospital.

At one point George told his wife he felt he was "slipping away, and if you don't start laying down on that horn, I'm not going to make it." She wished she could find a cop and get a police escort, but there were none to be seen.

What Mary did find though was a nearby filling station. She pulled in and looked around for help in getting George through the traffic. She quickly explained the situation to the station owner who assigned one of his attendants to aggressively drive the car for Mary and blow its horn continuously. This man also knew some shortcuts and was a near virtuoso at horn-blowing.

When George finally arrived at the hospital, he was still bleeding actively, but he was conscious. A review of the situation confirmed the impression that he most likely had a cardiac wound and that immediate repair was necessary as were blood transfusions and fluid replacement. George and I went to the operating room together.

As it turned out, Mary somehow had the presence of mind to bring along a current package of medical reports and X-rays from George's recently completed company physical exam. This material also contained an electrocardiogram which was nice to have, but it was of no help in making decisions about George's immediate need...surgical repair of his heart.

I opened the front of his chest as soon as he could be anesthetized. His heart was found to be compressed by a large collection of blood in the pericardium, the sack-like structure that contains and protects the heart. With the blood removed, a cut approximately two inches long became apparent in the front wall of the right ventricle, which is the part of the heart that pumps the venous blood flow through the lungs to become oxygenated. The cardiac wound in the right ventricle seemed to be the only immediate problem. The other surgeons and I exposed it and repaired it carefully with about five sutures. We protected the coronary arteries carefully, making sure not to interfere with the flow of blood through the coronary vessels supplying the heart muscle itself.

The other cardiac structures were intact, showing that the clipper blade had not passed completely through the heart but through the front heart wall only. None of the other chest contents including the lungs and major blood vessels were injured significantly. The rest of the heart including the left ventricle—the highest pressure pump—was beginning to perform better as his blood volume was replaced. George's blood pressure went from unobtainable to low, and then became normal. Having successfully fixed his bleeding heart and confirming there was no bleeding going on in George's chest, we implanted a temporary plastic drainage tube and closed the incision.

Once his fluids and blood volume were restored to a near normal level, George regained stability and awakened from his anesthesia without any problems. He received about six transfusions in all.

The whole heart muscle escaped any injury except for the right ventricular wound. The left ventricle, which is directly behind the right ventricle in the lower chest, was not involved. The right ventricular wound was not much different from a surgical incision, and the wound edges were clean and healthy in appearance. George was fortunate there was no injury to any of the other chest contents. He could easily have injured other parts of the heart or other organs, and he might well not have been able to survive.

George's progress to healing was interrupted only by a few days of benign pericarditis, inflammation of the sack that contains the heart. It responded well to treatment with appropriate medication and steroids. ("Benign" is not an accurate term for this condition, as I discovered years later when I had a bout of "benign" pericarditis following a pacemaker-insertion procedure. It was a revelation to me as to how much pain an attack of good old "benign" pericarditis could bring on.)

Of course, George made the front pages of all the local newspapers. Some of the faraway papers also carried a brief report of this falling-on-the-hedge clippers story. As a result, he received get-well cards from people he knew, but had not seen in years.

His postoperative course was smooth once the pericarditis was resolved, and George ended up enjoying his ten-day hospital stay. Once he got to the point where his life was out of danger, he gave a lot of praise to everybody concerned with getting his heart fixed. George came to understand that he had a wife with a lot of grit who was largely responsible for having things ready to fix his situation. He was anxious to give her full credit for her part in getting him to the hospital and said, as quoted in one of his newspaper interviews, "My wife, the way she kept herself together during that drive...she's a brick!"

The story does not quite end there. I was eating lunch with a group of doctors in the office building a few weeks later when a young internist asked me just how I went about deciding on a fair price to charge for what was obviously a life-saving procedure, as in George's case. Something made me tell him with the straightest face I could muster that my usual method was to interview the patient's boss and get an estimate of the patient's value to his company as well as how fast his boss thought he would be expected to move up in salary and bonus. I told the internist I then would estimate the effects of inflation and settle on a quarterly payment amounting between twenty and twenty-five percent of his expected earnings for the rest of his life, but without any interest if all the payments were made timely.

The look on the internist's face was something to behold until he caught on with the rest of the lunchers that this was not really the way I set my fees. Sometimes, now and again, I think it might not be such a bad idea after all.

At any rate, I last talked to George a couple of years afterwards when he called wanting some advice about one of his children. I found him to be doing quite well.

The first report of a successful repair of the heart with penetrating cardiac trauma was published in 1902, when a cardiac stab wound was surgically repaired. Our friend Dr. Boerhaave wrote in the early eighteenth century that all penetrating cardiac wounds were fatal. Current estimates are that about twenty-five percent of trauma deaths are due to cardiac trauma and about ten percent of gunshot injuries involve the heart. Recovery rates from cardiac trauma are now in the thirty to fifty percent range with aggressive diagnosis and treatment. The best diagnostic information for the presence or absence of cardiac trauma is the echocardiogram, while the EKG and pericardiocentesis are of little use because of the false negatives and false positives that result.

In my opinion, a large measure of credit in this case should go to George himself who devised a way to keep himself from bleeding out on the way to the hospital, and to Mary for getting things organized and under way to the emergency room. The service station employee also deserves commendation for being such a talented and willing horn player so Mary could get George to the hospital.

Obviously, there are many ways this story could have turned out differently, but this is really the way it all came down, for which George is grateful.

My final advice to George was: 1) find the missing electric shears, 2) give up trimming hedges altogether, or 3) get a taller wife. Since he seemed unlikely to find a wife who was both tall and extra efficient like Mary, I thought either solution number one or two would work best in this particular situation.

As it turned out, George promised Mary he would not use the hedge clippers ever again. He stated he had clipped his last hedge, and he would bring in an expert to do the job from then on. He also came to believe there are simpler and less dangerous ways to figure out that hedge clipping should be left to the experts, and that there is some virtue in watching sports on TV on weekend afternoons.

A Surprise Going-Away Present from Delores

Delores had always considered herself to be a healthy young woman. Her only significant health problem was as a result of an automobile accident in 1959, when she was diagnosed with a large collection of blood in her left chest. This issue worried those who were taking care of her, she remembered, but no specific diagnosis was made nor was any treatment carried out. Except for the birth of her two children, Delores had not been hospitalized since.

According to the information available, Delores had not suffered any other known specific serious internal injuries or broken bones as a result of the accident. She was living an active life without any pain or disability.

Although she was asymptomatic, she was given a chest X-ray as part of a routine periodic physical assessment by her internist in April of 1967, a little over seven years after the automobile accident. The X-ray revealed an intriguing abnormality. There was a swelling and enlargement in the thoracic aorta shadow on the left side of Delores' chest.

The aorta is the largest artery in the body. It takes oxygenated blood pumped from the heart via various branches to all the rest of the body. The enlargement, or aneurysm, in Delores' aorta was in the part of the aorta just beyond a major branch that takes blood to the left arm, near the beginning of the descending thoracic aorta.

This is also the area where the aorta is relatively free of small branches but makes a somewhat sharp curve towards the spine in its course to the lower extremities. It is a common area for injury to the aorta in sudden deceleration instances such as a head-on automobile crash or a fall from a height, even a fall from a horse. The aorta can become torn in this sort of an injury, sometimes actually torn in half, and there is an immediate fatal result in about eighty percent of the cases.

The type of accident involving violent deceleration brings about such a tear in part because of the configuration of the thoracic aorta and the stresses that are generated as the aorta goes around its arch and the flow of blood changes direction by about 180 degrees over a fairly short distance. Occasionally, the tissues surrounding the aorta, though not really strong at all compared to the healthy aorta itself, may be able to contain most of the bleeding that results from the aortic injury. The aorta may be able to continue to perform its job pretty well, except that usually the containing tissues will slowly stretch and weaken over time, sometimes over a period of several years.

As a usual course, the aneurysm—the swollen and thinned-out portion of the injured aorta—slowly enlarges over time. There may be intermittent pain in the chest for years as the tissues in the aneurysm wall stretch and the aneurysm gradually enlarges. And then, the aneurysm may quite suddenly give way at the point of injury and rupture days, weeks, months or even years following the initial injury.

Survival of the patient is most unlikely when this happens, as you might imagine, because the patient loses a large amount of blood quite suddenly. Even if the condition is known to exist, when the aneurysm suddenly ruptures, there is not enough warning to allow for the necessary preparations to be made to deal with the situation surgically, and the victim bleeds out within a few minutes.

Surgical repair of the aneurysm is the treatment of choice whenever this problem is detected. As in Delores' case, the diagnosis is frequently made from the appearance of the aneurysm on a chest X-ray taken for some other reason.

The earliest description of a traumatic aneurysm was made by Andreas Vesalius (1514–1564) in 1557, and the case he first described was due to a horseback-riding injury. Somehow there were no causative auto accidents blamed at that time largely, perhaps, because there were no automobiles yet. The automobile is now by far the cause of most instances of the problem. But in the case described by Vesalius, the patient had a fatal secondary rupture of the aorta about two years after what was thought to be the responsible injury, which was brought about from an accidental fall off a horse.

This is apparently what happened to the famous Western scout, frontiersman and Indian fighter Kit Carson. His primary aortic injury was thought to have been the result of his falling out of the saddle several years before his death from a secondary aortic disruption. Carson had intermittent chest pain for several years before he died, which might well have been related to changes in his blood pressure. With added stress on the thin tissues making up the wall of the aneurysm, his blood pressure might have risen as a result of his active lifestyle and his high level of physical activity.

The behavior and stability of the traumatic aneurysm over time seems to depend to a large extent on the avoidance of arterial hypertension (high blood pressure) among other factors.

With Delores' history of the automobile accident, the resulting bleeding in the left chest, and the clear X-ray evidence of a swollen aorta, it seemed highly likely that the aorta had been torn in her 1959 accident but had somehow held together completely undetected for over seven years. This impression was confirmed by an aortagram, a series of X-rays taken while a contrast material is injected into the aorta through a small plastic tube. This plastic tube is inserted through a needle and positioned so that the exact location of the aneurysm can be determined.

The appearance on X-ray of the contrast material flowing into Delores' aneurysm definitively confirmed the presence of an apparently stable traumatic aortic aneurysm. Delores' aneurysm was seen clearly just at the typical location for these injuries to occur. The aorta swings sharply downward toward the diaphragm at this point, and it is by far the most frequent site of injury due to a sudden deceleration type of insult.

Because of the significant enlargement of the aorta, there was obviously an ongoing threat to her life. I strongly recommended immediate, elective surgical repair of the aorta now that its presence was known and before it underwent a spontaneous secondary rupture. Delores and her family were made aware of a fairly long list of possible complications, and she was admitted to the hospital on an urgent basis.

Since the flow of blood through the aorta must be stopped while carrying out a lengthy repair, it is necessary to have a bypass apparatus set up. This allows the patient's blood to be pumped and circulated to the body during surgery while ensuring an unhurried dissection of the aorta and the aneurysm.

The bypass technique is pretty similar to the one used for open-heart surgery, except that it is performed by taking the blood out of the left atrium, where it has been already oxygenated by going through the lungs, and pumping it back into one of the large arteries in the groin area. From there blood can flow up the arterial system in retrograde fashion to help nourish the body during the actual repair of the aneurysm itself. The patient is anticoagulated during the use of bypass technology.

The operative procedure on Delores was carried out successfully, and the partially disrupted aorta was repaired using a segment of a plastic cloth-like tubular graft. This material was sutured to the injured aorta in such a way that a full-strength aorta was restored, and the injured portion was removed. Delores certainly seemed to be one of the fortunate twenty percent of patients whose tissue around the site of an aortic tear was strong enough to contain the bleeding as the traumatic aneurysm developed. Ordinarily, that tissue is quite flimsy.

Great care was taken to do as small an amount of dissection as possible to minimize the chances of inadvertent injury to the small arteries which nourish the spinal cord, avoiding any injury which might result in spinal cord malfunction.

Delores was young and healthy and tolerated the surgery well. She was kept in the intensive care area for several days for close observation.

She had a husky voice for a brief period of time postoperatively. This was thought to be due to pressure during surgery on one of the small nerves which passes beside and loops around the aorta in the area of the aneurysm on its way to the vocal cord on the left side of the larynx.

Delores' voice came back to normal on about the second day postoperative, and she got along quite well for the rest of her ten-day stay in the hospital. She did need to be on blood-thinning medication for a while because of a suspected small blood clot which probably formed in her leg and went to one lung (pulmonary embolus). But with her voice working well and her blood-thinning medication regulated, Delores was able to increase her activities satisfactorily at home and was seen in my office on a number of occasions as her progress continued. She was able to stop the blood thinner when she reached full activity level and had no more blood clots.

Delores was thought to be essentially healed from her injury and the surgery and to be pretty much as good as new within a few weeks. I felt good about her result and was delighted that she had gotten along so well and did not have to worry anymore about having a traumatic aortic aneurysm.

Several months after Delores' surgery, I began preparing for a presentation I was to make at the January 1980 meeting of the Rocky Mountain Trauma Society in Colorado. I was to discuss other cases in my surgical experience similar to Delores' traumatic aortic aneurysm.

I was at the Atlanta airport just prior to boarding a flight to the meeting when, out of the blue, Delores paged me on the old airport paging system. I returned her call on the telephone, and she told me she was having serious suicidal thoughts. She was distraught with fear that she would commit suicide unless she got help right away. I was not sure I could get in touch with a psychiatrist who would be able and willing to meet her obvious immediate requirements for attention and psychiatric care, but clearly that took precedence over my flight plans and conference presentation.

Fortunately, I quickly was able to get through to a psychiatrist friend of mine. To my surprise and delight, he assured me he would take care of everything for me and for Delores. I was much impressed by my friend's willingness to be available on such short notice, and it changed my opinion of psychiatrists and customer service completely. He was willing to step right in to a touchy situation and do a lot of what I thought were extra things because Delores really needed immediate attention.

With Delores in capable hands, I left for the conference as planned, and while there, I received encouraging telephone reports of her further progress and improvement. Comfortably assured of her well-being, I admit I did take time to enjoy a few trips down the ski slopes after the trauma meeting was over.

Thanks to the effective treatment provided by my psychiatrist friend, Delores got over her suicidal ideation in pretty short order, and she soon regained her previous mental health status.

Sam and the Long, Long, Long Tunnel

I met Sam in the middle of the night in Shepherd Center, a world-renowned spinal rehabilitation center in Atlanta. He was a teenage traumatic quadriplegic—meaning all four limbs were paralyzed—as a result of a recent accident in which his neck was broken and his spinal cord was crushed.

Sam's ability to breathe was considerably impaired due to the paralysis of the muscles involved in breathing air into and out of his lungs. Consequently, he was being aided by mechanical ventilation and/or supplemental oxygen as required, and he had tracheostomy and endotracheal tubes in place.

The tracheostomy is a metal tube placed in the trachea, the main air pipe, through a small incision in the front of the lower neck. It allowed comfortable augmentation of Sam's air exchange, reducing the difficulty he had breathing adequately and removing secretions from his airway. His oxygenation needs were checked frequently using an oximeter, and the oxygen level and mechanical breathing assistance were adjusted frequently as indicated.

At Shepherd Center, the hope was to gradually wean Sam from his dependence on the respiratory support. Although he was making slow, but steady progress with his rehabilitation, he still needed considerable respiratory support. Nonetheless, the expectation was that in time, he would recover some of his muscle strength and that he would be able to breathe on his own. For the moment though, Sam was highly dependent on machine-assisted ventilation to ensure he was getting adequate oxygenation.

Shepherd Center is next door to Piedmont Hospital, a large general hospital that serves many of the needs of the spinal center patients including anesthesia services, operating rooms, recovery areas and the like. The two buildings are connected by an underground tunnel several hundred feet long with zigs and zags and a fairly gentle, but steady uphill slope.

Sam was a patient I had never seen before. One of the spinal center nurses called me asking for immediate help when, in the middle of the night, Sam suddenly and unexpectedly began to bleed seriously into, through and around his tracheostomy tube. There was no problem making a diagnosis.

Erosion through the adjacent wall of one of the main arteries (the brachiocephalic artery) from the heart to the head, right arm and upper body just below the base of the neck by a tracheostomy tube is a serious complication. It is variously reported in the surgical literature as happening in about 0.7 percent of all the patients who have tracheostomy procedures[3].

I asked the nurse to alert the operating room at Piedmont to get ready for a chest operation quickly and to get anesthesia help, instruments and other equipment we would need. We discussed the quickest way to the operating room in the general hospital, and we all agreed the connecting tunnel was the way to go. That became the plan we would follow as soon as I could get there and we could get Sam on a stretcher.

Things did not look good for Sam. It was difficult for him to breathe adequately by means of a hand-squeezed bag connected to a portable oxygen tank, all the while keeping pressure on his lower neck to slow the bleeding as we aspirated and cleared the blood and secretions from his airway. This was difficult while he was in his bed. We knew it would be even more difficult to push him through the tunnel, keeping him oxygenated and slowing the bleeding as best we could.

We were certainly correct in our assumption that the trip would be difficult and a successful result uncertain at best. The staffing level at night for the spinal center was limited, and it ended up that a male nurse and I had to try to keep Sam alive and physically get him to the operating room so I could operate and hopefully stop the bleeding.

I rushed to Shepherd and looked over the situation. This helpful nurse and I got Sam onto a stretcher along with his oxygen supply and a portable suction machine with which to keep his airway free and unobstructed. We started through the uphill tunnel keeping Sam alive by applying hand pressure on his neck which diminished the bleeding considerably, trying to keep his airway clear of blood and pumping his lungs with oxygen while also pushing and guiding the stretcher.

We could have used at least two other helpers to accomplish the things Sam badly needed to have done, but there was no one else available. I was not sure any of us would get through to the end of the tunnel alive.

This was one of the most physically demanding activities I have ever had to perform on the job, and I believe if it had not been for the strong, young male nurse involved, we could not possibly have gotten to the end of that tunnel with a live patient.

We had no idea what Sam's blood pressure, pulse or any other vital signs were, but they couldn't have been any good. I decided it was just as well not to know.

The nurse and I finally got him to the operating room, but we were both at the end of our ability to function. We were joined there by some others including an anesthesiologist, a scrub nurse, and a surgical resident. We got busy transitioning immediately from a transport team to a surgical team. We were then able to open Sam's chest and find the brachiocephalic artery which was bleeding actively.

The only practical way to stop the bleeding under these circumstances is to ligate the artery just above and just below the source of the bleeding. This artery is one of the major ones and goes principally from the ascending aorta to the head and right arm. Since the brachiocephalic, or innominate, artery is one of the two major sources of blood flow to the brain, there is always the chance the brain may not be able to function normally after ligation of active bleeding. There is less of a chance of this kind of problem in a young person, but a chance nonetheless.

I felt there was really no choice, if we were going to be able to save Sam's life. And, indeed, Sam retained his mental function after the bleeding vessel was controlled by ligation.

I proceeded to expose the injured portion through an incision in the right upper chest and neck as soon as Sam was under anesthesia. The part of the innominate artery that had been eroded by the tracheostomy tube and was the cause of the bleeding was swiftly located and tied off above and below with a heavy-gage thread tie.

Sam was provided with a plastic endotracheal tube and it was carefully positioned to avoid pressure on any of the several large blood vessels in the neighborhood. With the bleeding stopped, we were able to replace his blood volume by transfusions.

Sam was transferred back to the spinal rehabilitation center from the general hospital several days later and resumed his care there. After a few weeks, during which he remained stable, Sam returned to his hometown hospital from which he had come originally.

Frankly, I was surprised we were able to keep Sam alive during the tunnel dash, but he did survive somehow and was not much the worse for wear as it turned out. The tunnel trip, hard enough on his panting and breathless transport team, had to have been unbelievably difficult for Sam.

This kind of surgical adventure shows it is not always just the surgical skills that may save the day–or night–as the case may be, but sometimes brute strength, stamina and endurance can be important too.

Sam's problem is thankfully much less likely to occur now. Newer models of tracheotomy tubes are a great deal less apt to erode nearby arteries. Babies and small children, though, are still subject to the erosion of blood vessels, but in lesser numbers than previously. A report in *Annals of Surgery* from 1976 stated that of the 137 cases of documented brachiocephalic artery erosion by a tracheotomy tube, only twenty-five percent of patients survive long term.

Sam was one of the lucky ones.

Joe Prepares for a Race with Cancer

Joe is one of my favorite people. You cannot help but appreciate his easy-going manner and the way he responds to challenges in a quiet, but effective way. When I was asked to see him professionally, he was a hard-working, forty-nine-year-old who ran long-distance races as a hobby.

He stayed in top physical shape and trained with ten or more mile runs several times a week. He had no fat on his frame, thanks to his fitness routine and marathon preparation. He was accustomed to following a training schedule which included frequent early morning, pre-workday runs.

Joe was used to good health, but he began to notice unusual fatigue after running his typical training exercise. In mid-December of 1982, he sought medical attention from his internist who was an excellent sub-specialist in gastrointestinal diseases. After a battery of tests, Joe was found to have significant anemia, a low red blood-cell count and hemoglobin level in the blood. An extensive outpatient work-up with the usual additional lab work and X-rays could not locate the cause.

Entirely by happenstance, when Joe was in the local
hospital X-ray department for a chest film, he encountered
a radiologist who was working on a research study of the
possible value of an esophagram in investigating the cause of
anemia in patients. Joe agreed to have such an examination
done, and the radiologist performed the procedure as Joe drank
a small amount of liquid contrast material. When the test was
completed, Joe went on about his business feeling secure his
esophagus was okay.

In February of 1983, just a couple of months later, Joe
again was at the same X-ray department, and, again, the
same radiologist happened to be there. He asked Joe if he
could make another esophagram. This time, there turned
out to be a significant change in the appearance of the lower
esophagus, and the suspicion pointed to cancer. This led Joe's
gastroenterologist-internist to carry out an esophagoscopy,
in which a flexible endoscope is passed down the esophagus
through the mouth. This allows a careful inspection of
the esophagus and upper stomach, and using special
instrumentation, biopsies of the esophagus can also be done.

In the lower part of Joe's esophagus there was a tumor which
only partially narrowed his esophagus and had not yet made for
any swallowing difficulty, the common symptom that usually
leads to the diagnosis of an esophageal problem. Multiple

biopsies were taken from the area of Joe's suspected tumor. The subsequent microscopic tissue examination of these biopsies revealed a definite cancer growing in Joe's lower esophagus. The appearance of the tumor suggested it was relatively small and fairly superficial. Thanks to the change picked up so nicely by the volunteer esophagrams, the tumor seemed to have been diagnosed at an unusually early stage in its development.

The important role played by the radiologist, who just happened to be at the right place at the right time for Joe and who was primarily responsible for the early diagnosis in Joe's case, cannot be overemphasized. Much of the credit for my having the opportunity to operate on what was really the earliest diagnosed esophageal cancer in my experience goes to him and to Joe's gastroenterologist-internist as well.

Esophageal cancer is among those human cancers with the worst prognosis and is among the most difficult of all cancers to cure. Although about twenty to thirty percent of the cancers of the esophagus are localized when they are discovered, the five-year survival rate is less than five percent. It tends to spread beyond the esophagus early in its development and is aggressively invasive. It is commonly diagnosed only after it has started to cause partial obstruction of the esophagus. By then it may have invaded neighboring tissues and/or spread to other areas of the body.

In Joe's case, a careful work-up—including more X-rays, lab tests and repeated physical exams—was given to pick up any evidence of cancer spread beyond the area which had been biopsied. Those tests did not show any signs of cancer-spread or metastasis.

There are those who feel the esophagus is not an organ designed to be operated upon, for there is a long list of serious complications which may ensue following attempts to remove these cancers surgically. These complications are in addition to the considerable uncertainty and difficulty in being able to remove all of the cancer surgically.

I knew Joe and his wife socially prior to these events, but I had never seen him as a patient until called in to address the management of his lower esophageal cancer. I proposed a surgical removal of the cancer with use of part of the upper stomach brought up into the chest to reestablish continuity of the gastrointestinal tract.

We discussed the serious nature of this surgery and the possible complications, but we also faced the lack of any other treatment with any real chance of success. Even if the cancer could be successfully removed, Joe might be subjected to some significantly unpleasant changes in his eating habits and enjoyment which are occasionally difficult to live with, including heartburn and decreased stomach capacity. Whether or not these kinds of problems are important and lasting difficulties after esophageal resection is impossible to predict ahead of time with any certainty.

Joe carried out his own research on esophageal cancer, using books and journals he had access to in various hospital libraries. He became quite knowledgeable. After due consideration, we all agreed that surgical removal would give the best and really only chance for success in curing the cancer in spite of the difficulties and possibility of complications or spread of the cancer.

We scheduled his surgery for a Monday morning at 7:30 and arranged for him to be admitted to the hospital the day before. Orders were written to prepare him for the surgery, and these were carried out as usual including shave and prep, pre-op medications and the like.

Under general anesthetic, the surgery went smoothly and was carried out in the usual way for this type of procedure. I worked in conjunction with an abdominal surgeon who concentrated on the preparation and management of much of the abdominal portion of the operation. I had the job of removing the cancer-bearing part of the esophagus, which amounted to just about the lower half of that organ. The upper portion of the stomach was then brought through the diaphragm and reattached to the remaining part of the esophagus up in the chest. Hopefully, that would allow Joe to swallow as normally as possible once he was healed.

Two surgeons working simultaneously allows a procedure to be done much more quickly than if done by a single surgeon. Equally important, it cuts down on the amount of time the patient is under anesthesia.

Joe spent a few days in the intensive care unit and remained in stable condition throughout the early phases of recovery. There were no problems whatever with any of the potential difficulties other than a small, temporary pancreatic fluid fistula (wound drainage) that closed spontaneously within a few weeks.

Joe was in the hospital for about two weeks altogether. When he began to eat, he started with multiple small meals, gradually becoming comfortable with fewer and larger meals until he was finally eating three square meals a day plus a bedtime snack. He soon resumed his running and exercise program and returned to his pre-operative weight of about 143 pounds, up from 132 pounds post-op.

Even though his progress was excellent, I somehow got the feeling during some of his postoperative visits to my office that there was something Joe had not told me. Although I was extremely pleased with his recovery in every way, I pressed him to come clean and fill me in on anything he felt he might ought to tell me.

After some hemming and hawing, he confessed he had come to a preoperative decision to do anything and everything he could think of to help with his healing and being cured of his disease. He decided he should present his body for the surgery in the best condition possible to be better able to heal rapidly and completely.

He had the idea that his body would be in its best shape only if he were to run about ten miles just before the operation. And so, he put on his running gear early on the Monday morning of surgery way before dawn and sneaked out of his hospital room, then out of the hospital. He ran ten miles, sneaked back into his room, showered and felt he had accomplished the aim of having his body at its peak of readiness for the surgery.

Nobody saw him leave his room, run or return. He told no one what he planned to do or that he had actually done the ten-mile run.

Joe was in no way surprised that he got along so beautifully after the surgery and avoided almost all of the many possible complications inherent in the type of surgery he had. This kind of success and recovery from the surgery was, after all, just what he expected and the reason he felt compelled to do the ten-mile run. It has been likewise no surprise to him that he has been cured of this dangerous cancer now for over two decades.

I have thought a lot about what I would have done had I known about Joe's ten-mile, preparatory run, and, repeatedly, I have been glad I was not aware of it. The anesthesiologist might well have refused to put him to sleep or the hospital might have prevented his having any surgery in its operating rooms. I would certainly have had a question as to whether to go ahead as planned with the surgery. And so, I do not know what might have happened if Joe had been caught sneaking in or out of the hospital, but I was glad he had not been caught and also glad, in retrospect, that I was not aware of this kind of preparation for the surgery. I am really not sure whether I would have postponed the operation, but, in any case, it would have been a difficult and bothersome decision, and I am glad I did not have to face it.

With all of the changes in the way hospitals are now built and staffed, and with present-day security in place, it seems unlikely that anyone could sneak undetected in and out of the hospital as Joe did on that early Monday morning in 1983. Most admissions to hospitals for surgery are now taking place on the day of surgery anyhow.

As far as I am concerned, Joe got along so smoothly after the surgery that it is hard to argue he did anything he shouldn't have. The fact that he is apparently cured of so serious and difficult a problem, now some twenty-five years after his operation, is a compelling argument. Maybe a ten-mile run should be a required preoperative exercise for all patients in the future if it can provide this kind of splendid outcome. I would not argue against it at all, but I have not encountered any other patient who has gone this far to prepare for a major operative procedure. Joe has continued to get along exceedingly well without any hints of recurrent cancer. He returned to work in March of 1983 and also ran in the 10K Peachtree Road Race on the Fourth of July that year.

Most unfortunately, Joe had a severe accidental injury to the nerves serving his left arm and shoulder about six years ago in a bicycle crash. He had two major reconstructive orthopedic procedures on his arm and shoulder which were only partially successful. And, ultimately, Joe's injury forced him to retire from his work, which he could no longer perform one-handed.

He has moved to a neighboring area on the Georgia coast, and we see each other from time to time at computer club meetings, art shows and the like. He spends his time helping his wife manage her business and doing volunteer work in the community. He is one of the examples I use to help explain to medical students some of the joys of surgery, and I get a big lift every time I see him.

Joe enjoyed running in the Boston Marathon in the mid-eighties, and he ran in various local long-distance races until about three or four years ago. Around the age of seventy, he stopped running and gave up on competing in long races.

I recently spent some time with Joe in exploring the circumstances of his treatment and care. He kindly discussed his side of the experiences, which are interesting as well as unique. Just finding a twenty-five year survivor of esophageal cancer to talk to is difficult to impossible, especially one who is so articulate and who has informed himself so well in the particulars of this disease.

His advice to others who need major kinds of surgery is to pay close attention to nutrition and to match exercise levels to food intake levels in order to maintain an ideal weight. He also advises use of the information available on the internet or in print. He found the journals produced by Sloan Kettering to be especially helpful to him in learning about the esophagus and esophageal cancer. My own observation has been that Joe's positive attitude, in spite of some really tough problems, was extremely helpful, as was the close support provided by his family.

During his race against cancer and his recovery from the bicycle accident, Joe came to recognize his own vulnerability, and he has adjusted to that realization. He is a remarkable example of adaptation to the vicissitudes he has had to face, and he has shown others how to deal with whatever problems come along.

Joe represents the ideal patient. He is certainly an important part of my group of special patients because of the joy he and the others have provided me in working with them.

Brian & Fred

HOW DID THAT HAPPEN?

Brian and Fred experienced similar and unusual cancerous tumors which arose in the skin and then invaded other organs. Malignant melanoma is a most difficult cancer to cure. It does not respond well to any of the available chemotherapy agents, and it tends to spread early anywhere within the body and recurs at the primary site to reinvade local tissues there.

The primary location of Brian's melanoma was in the skin of his ear. It then reappeared in his brain and finally became evident in his lungs. Fred had a primary in the skin of his forehead followed by multiple areas of metastases to both lungs and then brain involvement.

Both Brian and Fred were able to have their brain tumors removed and their neurological symptoms completely relieved by capable neurosurgery. In fact, they actually shared the same neurosurgeon. I was called in for the lung part.

The patient Brian
Brian is a professional artist and does wonderful things in various media. I have known him as a patient and a friend for

almost thirty years. When he was my patient, Brian recalled that in 1953 as a seventeen year old, he experienced bad cases of sunburn while working a summer job shoveling coal from railroad cars. Because he almost always faced the same direction as he worked, the right side of his face and especially his right ear were repeatedly sunburned.

In 1970 at age 34, Brian was diagnosed by biopsy with primary metastatic melanoma in the ear. It was removed surgically in radical fashion. Cancer-free margins were reported by the pathologist in Pennsylvania where Brian was living. Then in the spring of 1977, about seven years after the primary melanoma had been removed, Brian suddenly began to have loss of control of his right leg and arm and noted that he had trouble typing because his fingers did not behave properly.

He rushed home from a European trip to be seen by a neurologist and was found to have a brain tumor as the cause of his difficulties. He underwent a craniotomy and removal of what proved to be metastatic malignant melanoma. Brian made a satisfactory recovery with full return of his motor skills and his typing abilities.

During the work-up to diagnose his brain tumor, a right lung lesion was seen on Brian's chest X-ray, but it did not seem to be advancing or enlarging. Over the next eighteen months, though, the lung lesion showed through X-ray to be slowly increasing in size, and I was asked to see Brian about the advisability of removing the lesion.

I felt a resection of the lung lesion made sense in this unusually lethargic melanoma. As far as could be determined, the brain was free of any recurrence. And so, in January of 1979 operative removal of the lung mass was carried out. The removed tissue was confirmed as being a metastatic melanoma.

Except for an operative procedure by the neurosurgeon to encourage proper healing of the craniotomy area of the skull, Brian has not had any further treatment, and there has been no evidence of any recurrence of the melanoma over a period now of about thirty-plus years.

The Patient Fred

I have known Fred since our grammar school days, longer than I have known any other of these patients about whom I have written. We grew up in the same neighborhood, he being a couple of years older. Although I knew him, his manifest seniority in age did not permit him to acknowledge that anyone about twenty months younger than he was even alive.

Over the years, Fred went to law school and became a successful lawyer. Around age fifty-eight, he became concerned about something on the skin of his forehead. A biopsy by a dermatologist proved the concern to be malignant melanoma. Fred underwent an appropriate radical wide removal of the forehead cancer, and the examination of the radically excised forehead skin showed no cancer at the margins of the resection.

Fred had no chemotherapy or other treatment except for regular periodic exams and follow-up X-rays. Though he continued to be without symptoms, a chest X-ray administered during a routine physical exam revealed several tumor-like nodules about the size of marbles in each of Fred's lungs.

Although Fred was asymptomatic and had a completely negative exam except for the chest X-ray, the chances were thought to be greatly in favor of either spread of the melanoma to the lungs and/or the development of some other kind of cancer. The decision was then made to remove one or more of the tumor nodules surgically from the lungs so that the correct diagnosis would be certain. From there the most effective treatment could be identified, particularly if a new and different cancer were present.

On Valentine's Day of 1986, I carried out the pulmonary surgery using a procedure called a sternal split, a vertical incision through the sternum. This incision was chosen to provide access to both lungs. Since the tumor nodules were small and easy to remove through the sternal split, all of them—about a half-dozen all together, including some from each lung—were removed. At that point, there were no nodules remaining in either lung big enough to feel or see in the open chest. On pathological examination, all of those removed nodules from the lungs were found to be metastatic malignant melanoma.

Fred remembers that one of his daughters fainted in the recovery room when she went in to see her dad for the first time postoperatively. He also remembers having his chest tubes removed, as most patients do, and also being a little slow getting off the ventilator in the early postoperative period. His recovery in the hospital was generally smooth, and he got along well after the lung surgery for several months.

Then, while on a trip to London, Fred began having serious loss of balance and severe headaches. He returned home as quickly as possible.

A new, small tumor mass was found in the cerebellum, the part of the brain responsible for equilibrium and balance, among other things. His symptoms and findings fit a presumptive diagnosis again of metastatic disease from the malignant melanoma, and it explained the symptoms and findings of his serious intracranial problems.

Again, there were no other locations where any suspicion of additional metastases existed outside of the skull. Because of his pressing symptoms, the localized nature of the recurrence, and the lack of any other effective treatment, a craniotomy was carried out by his excellent neurosurgeon. The areas of metastatic melanoma were removed.

Fred made another rapid and successful recovery from the craniotomy and became asymptomatic in short order, regaining his balance and his equilibrium and getting rid of the severe headaches.

To the amazement of his friends, family and physicians, Fred has remained well to this day with no additional treatment of any kind, and there has not been any indication other than his surgical scars that he has ever had metastatic melanoma.

Surviving Malignant Melanoma–How Did That Happen?
Brian and Fred overcame malignant melanoma with lung and brain metastases without chemotherapy. They represent unexpected and most unusual outcomes for malignant melanoma, outcomes I have seen only in these two patients in my entire surgical career. As of this writing, Brian has been cancer-free for thirty-two years and Fred, for twenty-five years. How did that happen?

There is no easy answer as to how or why these two patients were able to overcome this advanced state of cancer invasion. Perhaps it was because their primary cancers were in such prominent and visible locations, bringing them to diagnosis and treatment earlier than the same cancer in a less visible, more undetectable location. And, while there was subsequent metastatic spread of the cancer to both the lungs and the brain, there was no recurrence of malignancy at either of their primary sites.

The decision to remove all of Brian's cerebellar metastatic brain nodules and all of Fred's palpable and visible lung tumors were additional keys to the unexpected success and long-term freedom from what is generally a fatal outcome.

My only other idea of a plausible explanation as to why Brian and Fred have achieved this apparent complete recovery from a really wicked and widespread cancer is that probably the tumor load, through surgery, became small enough to enable their own inherent cellular and molecular bodily defense mechanisms to overcome whatever residual cancer may have been present. Research in this area might be useful in deciding how to treat other similar patients. Something certainly seems to have spontaneously wiped out what must have been additional, undiagnosed microscopic cancer metastases which were likely present in unknown locations but were too small to be evident to the testing methods then available.

For Brian and Fred, the decades of apparent freedom from this kind of cancer is not an expected result, but it is excellent evidence that unexpected things do happen. Both of these patients remain free of any signs or symptoms, living productive and useful lives. Indeed, both patients' ability to overcome this invasive, mean and ugly cancer certainly borders on the miraculous.

CHAPTER FOUR

The Surgeon

As I write this, I am now approaching eighty years of age. I practiced surgery and was involved with resident training for about forty-seven years.

My retirement in 1988 gave me the opportunity to be a full-time maker and designer of furniture, something I had avoided during the practice years because I thought I could do better surgery with a full set of fingers on each hand. My wife and I were building a vacation/retirement house, and my homemade furniture mostly met with approving responses from her.

I was especially pleased with a display case I made to house my collection of used, early cardiac pacemakers. I had imagined this piece would stand in a prominent location in our new home and would show in a graphic way the progress made in the design and construction of pacemakers over a period of about twenty years. In addition, I reasoned, it would be a handy conversation starter.

Needless to say, my display case ended up instead in a remote bedroom corner, and I have to get special approval from my wife for it to be seen by any visitors. She has assured me it is the contents and not the case itself she objects to. You see, the design of pacemakers, especially in the early years, was somewhat short on aesthetics. The scramble to get the devices on the market meant manufacturers were concerned almost exclusively with functionality rather than with the looks of the product.

About a year or so after retirement, having designed and made furniture to my heart's content, I accepted a part-time position as the medical director for the Georgia Department of Corrections. It was one of those temporary jobs that managed to last two years while a full-time replacement was found, and it was both interesting and challenging.

The sudden appearance of HIV/AIDS and its rapid increase among the prisoners required immediate decision-making. On the line was the question of how and by whom—whether by general medical officers or by infectious disease specialists—it would be treated in the prison system. My feeling was that it would have to be handled mainly by the general medical officers because of the rate at which it was increasing.

My principal contributions as the medical director were to provide education for the staff physicians about HIV and to recruit medical and surgical specialists as part-time staff physicians for the prison system. Some of the doctors I knew who wanted to keep doing some limited clinical work after retirement were attracted to this, and they were enormously helpful.

My most favorite and enjoyable part-time and post-retirement activity, though, was as a field staff site visitor for the Accreditation Council for Graduate Medical Education. My participation in this most interesting activity was an enjoyable retirement activity, and I worked at it for fifteen years until the travel situation degenerated after the 9/11 attack.

The ACGME gig was a marvelous opportunity to travel about the country visiting teaching hospitals and university residency training programs—mostly, but not exclusively, surgical. My job was to obtain information that became the basis for the decision as to accreditation and to facilitate program repair when that was needed.

The site-visit process was based on a full day of interviews with residents, administrators, department chairmen, faculty members, hospital CEOs and program directors, followed by an inspection of the facilities. Afterwards, I wrote a twenty- to thirty-page report which allowed the program evaluation committee to make a valid accreditation decision.

The process was well organized and effective. New ideas were encouraged and tried. Special attention was devoted to troubled programs and programs with frequent leadership changes.

As a site visitor I was provided with a wide view of the training process across the country and given a chance to talk with trainees and educators at all levels. Based on those visits and conversations, judgment was made as to the future direction of post-graduate training, especially in surgery and the surgical specialties.

These contacts were of a different content and order of magnitude from those in the earthier and more direct world of state prisons. Both, though, allowed a wide view of the status of American surgery and the increasing diminution of the popularity of surgery as a career field for medical students.

And that is exactly why I have written this book.

About a half-minute of internet research gives 641,000 responses to the subject line "shortage of surgeons," and that is for both developed as well as undeveloped countries. A 2006 study conducted at the University of California shows surgical demand is on the rise because of an increasingly aging population in the United States. The *Chattanooga Times Free Press* reports "...a shortage of surgeons and physicians in general that is coming on like a freight train in this country."

A United States veterans hospital is said to have an eighteen-month backlog of some surgeries. Surgeons in San Antonio are thought to be shying away from trauma-call duty. In a hospital in Wales, kidney transplants have been halted for lack of surgeons.

The Australasian College of Surgeons and other learned colleges are being blamed for their monopoly control over surgical training and the choice of surgeons-to-be. *USA Today* has stated that lawsuits are principally behind the shortage of surgeons. In London, the fear is that British National Health System goals will not be met for lack of surgeons. The American Surgical Association reports there is a national defense problem when there is a shortage of surgeons in case there are terrorist attacks on our homeland.

The list goes on and on.

Surgeons need heart-warming events just like anyone else, and one thing is for sure: There will always be more "specials" waiting to reward surgeons-to-be as those of mine have rewarded me.

My Not-So-Secret Hope

In going through the review of cases for this book, I realize anew the great privilege it has been to be of definitive help to my patients. I am thankful for the opportunities to provide a successful outcome in some desperate situations.

I would again like to assert that I make no claim to possess special talents or wisdom, and that some other patients with similar problems did not fare as well as did the few I have written about in this work.

My not-so-secret hope in putting this material together is to encourage young people to consider the study of medicine and particularly surgery as a career.

The personal satisfaction that came from all of my patients, including those with unexpected results, is but just one indication of the opportunities provided in what I consider the joy of surgery.

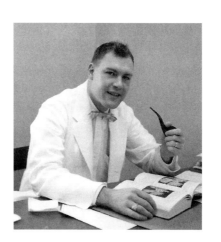

L. Newton Turk III, M.D.

College and Medical School – Emory University School of
    Medicine, BA, 1948; M.D. 1952

Internship in Surgery – Yale–New Haven Hospital, 1952-1953

USPHS Research Fellowship, Surgery – Yale School of
    Medicine, 1953-1954

US Air Force, Flight Surgeon – Walker AFB, 1954-1956

Resident in Surgery – Yale School of Medicine, 1956-1957

Surgical Fellowship – Harvard Medical School, Brigham and
    Women's Hospital, 1958

Chief Surgery Resident – Yale School of Medicine, 1959-1960

Fellow, American College of Surgeons

Fellow, American College of Chest Physicians

Diplomate of the American Board of Surgery

Diplomate of the Board of Thoracic Surgery

Past Faculty Appointments:
    Yale School of Medicine,
    Harvard Medical School,
    University of Kentucky College of Medicine,
    Emory University School of Medicine.

Past President, Georgia State Board of Medical Examiners

Former Board Member, Georgia Blue Cross Blue Shield

Past President, Medical Association of Atlanta

Past President, Medical Association of Georgia

Past President, Rocky Mountain Trauma Society

Former Board Member, International Foundation for Scholarly
Exchange

Former Committee Member on Thoracic Surgery, American
Thoracic Society

Visiting Professor of Surgery, Hospital Albert Schweitzer, Haiti

Medical Director, Georgia Department of Corrections

Site visitor, the Accreditation Council for Graduate Medical
Education, 15 years

In late 2010, our dad, Newton Turk, started showing signs of dementia, and at the publication of this book, he is in the throes of Alzheimer's. In his writing of the manuscript, long before Alzheimer's took its toll, he wrote, "I'd like to thank everybody who helped with this book. You know who you are." Concise, to the point, typical, but most especially, an indication of his tongue-in-cheek sense of humor. We always smile when we read that comment.

Dad's humor aside, we know he would want to thank the following people for their help in making this book a reality: Eliza Hunter, his granddaughter who visited him after her school day ended and helped him organize the material for this book; Corinne Adams, Dr. Pamela Battey, Dr. Molly Moye, Jim Spratt and Susan Thomas for their careful reading of the manuscript; Jeanne Potter, our editor, for her great support, encouragement, and knowledge; and David Laufer for his guidance and creativity.

To all the rest...*you know who you are.*

1. Sheldon GF. "Access to Care and the Surgeon Shortage–American Surgical Association Forum." *Annals of Surgery.* 252, 4 (2010): 582–590. (page 25)

2. Turk LN, Glenn WWL. "Cardiac Arrest: results of attempted cardiac resuscitation in 42 cases." *New England Journal of Medicine.* 251. (1954): 795–803. (page 44)

3. Jones JW, Reynolds M, Hewitt RL, Drapanas T. "Tracheo-innominate artery erosion: successful surgical management of a devastating complication." *Annals of Surgery*. 1976: 194–2004. (page 73)

Colophon

Unexpected Results
Set in the Bembo type family,
originally cut by Francesco Griffo around 1495,
and revived by the Monotype Corporation in 1929.
Chapter titles set in Deepdene Italic,
designed by Frederick Goudy in 1928
Printed on Mohawk Superfine.
Bound in Pearl Linen binding cloth by LBS.
Printed by Thomson Shore, Dexter, Michigan

Design by Susan Spratt and Gregor Turk
with assistance from David Laufer, Atlanta Georgia
Frontispiece illustration by Mark Andresen, Atlanta, Georgia.
Manufactured in USA